MW00512499

KETO DIET FOR BEGINNERS

Complete Beginner's Guide To The Ketogenic Diet
With Delicious And Easy Recipes To Lose Weight
And Eat Healthy Everyday

JULIE ARDEN

Copyright © 2018 Julie Arden

All rights reserved.

In no way is it legal to reproduce, duplicate, or transmit any part of this document in either electronic means or in printed format. recording of this publication is strictly prohibited and any storage of this document is not allowed unless with written permission from the publisher. all rights reserved. The information provided herein is stated to be truthful and consistent, in that any liability, in terms of inattention or otherwise, by any usage or abuse of any policies, processes, or directions contained within is the solitary and utter responsibility of the recipient reader. under no circumstances will any legal responsibility or blame be held against the publisher for any reparation, damages, or monetary loss due to the information herein, either directly or indirectly. Respective authors own all copyrights not held by the publisher. The information herein is offered for informational purposes solely, and is universal as so. the presentation of the information is without contract or any type of guarantee assurance. The trademarks that are used are without any consent, and the publication of the trademark is without permission or backing by the trademark owner. all trademarks and brands within this book are for clarifying purposes only and are the owned by the owners themselves, not affiliated with this document. The author wishes to thank 123RF / karandaev for the image on the cover.

TABLE OF CONTENTS

JULIE ARDEN

Introduction

Congratulations on purchasing *Keto Diet For Beginners: Complete Beginner's Guide To The Ketogenic Diet With Delicious And Easy Recipes To Lose Weight And Eat Healthy Everyday* and thank you for doing so. The ketogenic diet is a surefire way to lose weight while at the same time helping you to access previously untapped sources of energy that will help you to look and feel better than you have in years.

While the benefits are certainly worth it, taking the plunge with the keto diet can be tricky which is why the following chapters will discuss everything you need to know in order to get started on the right foot. First, you will learn all about the many benefits of the keto diet and why it is the weight loss solution you have been waiting for. Next, you will learn all about the types of foods you can expect to enjoy while following the keto diet as well as how to eat out while sticking to the diet. From there you will find additional tips for success as well as a 14-day meal plan to help you get you through the early days of the diet.

There are plenty of books on this subject on the market, thanks again for choosing this one! Every effort was made to ensure it is full of as much useful information as possible, please enjoy!

Chapter 1:
How the Keto Diet Affects Your Health

The ketogenic diet follows a low-carbohydrate, moderate-protein, and high-fat eating plan, that places the body in a state called "ketosis." This diet retrains the body to use fats as its primary source of energy, rather than carbohydrates. When a person eats something that is high in carbs, the body naturally turns it into two products: glucose and insulin. Any glucose that is not used up is essentially stored in our muscle tissue and liver.

Ketosis is a completely natural process that occurs when the body is starved of carbohydrates and begins producing ketones from breaking down fat in the liver.
Insulin is necessary for our bodies to stay healthy. However, extra carbs are not good for us. They cause excess weight gain in our mid-section and even cause us to become diabetic. Carbs, when broken down, are made of glucose and insulin. As long as we eat the right amount of carbs, we can maintain our insulin without overdoing the glucose, which is a derivative of sugar. Glucose is bad for our health and can cause excess fat and even acne. So, eliminating the glucose from our diets is a good option for everyone.

So, you may ask who is the keto diet best for? Well, that is simple. Everyone can benefit from the keto diet including athletes. Athletes use the keto diet to optimize their insulin with foods high in Omega-3 fatty acids. A keto diet is a great option for those that are paleo, vegan, and vegetarian, as well as those that are pescatarian. The great thing about the Keto diet is that you do not specifically have to eat meat. You just have to eat a high-fat, moderate-protein, and low-carb diet.

Benefits of the Keto Diet

The biggest benefit of the keto diet, you can really eat anything that you want. There are going to be some foods that you are going to want, to stay away from which will be discussed in a later chapter, but, that is just so that you are not placing too many carbs in your system. Other than that, you can eat anything and everything! How great is that?

Weight loss: This is probably the number one reason why people go on a keto diet. Indeed, with the power of ketosis, this diet appears to be the number one diet when it comes to burning fats. Once you are in ketosis, what other fat-burning plans do you need? It is already the optimal state for burning fat for fuel. If you really want to lose weight and make those tight abs appear, then you should definitely consider going on a keto diet. But, it doesn't just end there. The keto diet has many other benefits.

Improve blood pressure: Ketosis can also help with your blood pressure. Ketosis, in a word, causes you to pee – a lot. This means that your body requires a lot more water. However, in this heavier urination, you also shed a lot more electrolytes, meaning that your sodium levels can go down massively which will benefit your blood pressure.

The simple idea behind ketosis and the ketogenic diet is simply taking in fat as your main source of cholesterol. One may think that this seems counterintuitive to helping one's blood pressure and general health. However, it's quite the opposite. If you were to run lab tests after having a healthy ketogenic diet for six months, you would find that your lipid levels were higher, your bad cholesterol levels were lower, your good cholesterol levels were higher, and your blood pressure is lower and far more stable than it may have been before. In other words, your blood becomes a lot healthier – and so do you!

Increased mental focus and physical endurance: Unlike other diets that will leave you feeling weak and dizzy, the keto diet will make you feel incredibly energized. It will also give you increased mental focus that is unique only to those people who have experienced what it's like to be in a state of ketosis.

Although you might not feel this right away, you will definitely enjoy these benefits after your body has adjusted to the diet. Whether you are preparing for a competition or simply want to feel healthier and stronger, then the keto diet is for you. If you just want to enjoy having a clear mind and being able to think more effectively, then this diet can also be helpful. And, since the keto diet is something that you can use for an extended period, then you can enjoy these benefits (as well as other benefits) for a long period of time.

A common mistake is to give up and abandon the diet before your body can adjust to it. Before you even start out on a keto diet, you should make it clear to yourself that you will have to face some discomfort and challenges. However, if you stay strong and give yourself enough time to adjust, then you will soon experience and enjoy the full benefits offered by this diet.

Additional benefits
- Getting your body into the metabolic state of ketosis has been proven to have several positive physical effects.
- Bodies will develop a preference for using ketones as a source of fuel instead of glucose created by the consumption of carbs
- Lowers insulin, which promotes the release of growth hormones for healthy muscle building
- Suppresses hunger with the consumption of more protein
- Reduces insulin levels, allowing kidneys to rid themselves of excess sodium
- Body no longer holds onto excess water
- Reduction of fat molecules, a.k.a. triglycerides that contribute to heart disease
- Decrease in blood sugar levels
- Increase in good cholesterol (HDL)
- Natural, non-addictive treatment for brain disorders, such as epilepsy
- Treatment for metabolic syndrome
- A natural, less invasive cancer treatment by eliminating the sugary fuel that cancerous cells feed on

Risks on the Keto Diet

Like many things in life, the keto diet too has its pros and cons. Before you start on this diet, it's best to be aware of the potential risks to those just starting out. As with all diets, it is also a good idea to talk to your doctor about any changes you are planning to make to your diet, and what impact that might have on your health.

Muscle loss: As you lower your calorie intake, you need to be mindful of how many calories you are also burning. When the body runs out of stored fats for fuel, it will turn to burning muscle mass if it has to. If you plan on working out, you need to account for this in your dietary intake.

Development of ketoacidosis: If your level of ketones become too unbalanced, it may lead to the creation of this condition. This occurs when the pH levels in your blood decrease, thus allowing for an environment of high acidity, which can be extremely threatening to those that have conditions such as diabetes.

Nutrient deficiencies: Low-carb diets are lacking in micronutrients, such as iron, potassium, and magnesium. You will more than likely have to invest in taking quality multivitamins on daily basis.

Chapter 2:
Macros and How They Work Within the Keto Diet

As the ketogenic diet is based around the idea of maintaining ketosis, there are few traditional tricks when it comes to ensuring the process is as successful as possible. Instead, it is important to ensure that changing your eating habits doesn't disrupt the proper mixture of vitamins and nutrients from making it into your system. If you were not previously a healthy eater prior to adopting the keto diet then this is the perfect opportunity to start putting real thought into the foods you eat rather than simply eating the first thing that you find.

There are three main macronutrients (macros) that you are going to need to keep an eye on if you want your body to respond to your time in ketosis as effectively as possible. These include fats, proteins, and carbohydrates. For starters, in order to ensure that you remain in ketosis once you reach it, then you are going to want to focus on eating lots of fats, about 90 percent of which should be of the healthy variety. As long as this is the case then the other 10 percent can be anything you like and you will still come out with a net positive.

When it comes to lean protein, it is important to keep in mind that even the healthiest options out there are going to be 55 percent antiketogenic which means that you will need to keep a close eye on your consumption, especially when you are first making the transition to the keto diet. Finally, by this point, you should not be surprised by the revelation that carbohydrates are completely antiketogenic, no matter the specifics which means they need to be consumed very carefully. All told, each of your meals needs to be made up of about 70 percent healthy fat, 25 percent protein, and 5 percent carbs.

Foods to eat

Protein: You are going to want to keep your protein consumption to a tight 25 percent of your total caloric intake for the day which means it pays to be a little picky with your choices. For starters, you will need to stay away from non-organic options as not all proteins are going to automatically be good for you. In fact, many non-organic proteins are actually known to contain a host of bacteria, as well as harmful steroids, neither of which are going to do your body any favors. This is why it is so important to eat meat that is certified organic, locally grown and grass-fed.

When it comes to healthy protein, there are few more healthy options than fish as it contains several different healthy oils in addition to the right amount of lean protein. This is not the same for farm-raised fish, however, as they are typically much lower in healthier nutrients then their all-natural counterparts. Good choices when it comes to fish includes halibut, Mahi-Mahi, sardines, sole, tuna, snapper, catfish, salmon and anchovies. The same thing goes for shellfish include mussels, oysters, shrimp, crabs, and lobster. Red meat is also a viable alternative assuming the cut is lean in fat and that the animals were raised in an organic and grass-fed environment. Reasonable options in this arena include veal, lamb, venison and beef.

Poultry is another lean and healthy options as long as they are also raised in an organic and free-range environment. Poultry that is up for grabs includes chicken, turkey, goose, pheasant, and duck. Additionally, it is important to remember that eggs are always going to be a good source of lean protein. Organic and free-range eggs are even better. As long as it follows the general guidelines, all types of pork are also accessible. This doesn't include pre packaged bacon and sausage as it is typically chocked full of preservatives and sugars. While peanuts and soy beans both contain a decent amount of protein, it is important to severely limit your intake of them because they contain lots of carbohydrates as well.

Fats and oils: When it comes to ensuring that you are eating the right healthy fats each day you are going to want to pay special attention to omega 6 and omega 3 as you need an equal amount of both in order to remain healthy in the long term. Fish or fish oil supplements will help to keep your omega levels in balance. It is also important to ensure you keep your diet filled with both saturated and monosaturated fats. If you have a choice, you are going to want to aim for those that are chemically stable as this means they are healthy as well. Viable choices for these types of fats include things like coconut oil, avocado oil, grass-fed organic butter, and egg yolks.

Carbs: While you are only allowed a very small amount of carbs per day, this doesn't mean you can blow them all without giving them a second thought. Instead, it is important to use your carb allotment on healthy choices like dark, leafy green vegetables as these are going to have more nutrients per serving than any other alternative.

Vegetables that have a viable number of carbs when consumed in moderation includes things like kale, sprouts, garlic, cabbage, radishes, spinach, dill pickles, bok choy, broccoli, asparagus, cauliflower, chives, leeks, and cucumbers. However, if your favorite type of vegetable isn't on this list, that doesn't mean it is off limits completely, it only means that you are going to need to carefully track how much you consume to avoid making a costly mistake.

Dairy: When it comes to working to achieve ketosis for the very first time, you are going to want to avoid consuming dairy products while you are in the transition phase as doing so has the potential to create an immediate insulin spike that may be high enough to knock you out of ketosis completely. What's more, dairy contains both whey and casein which both contain enough protein to throw off your desired macros when not consumed sparingly.

While it is recommended that you abstain from dairy completely, if you must you will find the best options to be cream cheese, sour cream, cottage cheese, mascarpone cheese, whipping cream and whole milk to be the best options as long as they are all used sparingly. When it comes to most cheeses you can generally assume that a gram of cheese contains one gram of carbs.

Liquids: When it comes to vital parts of the keto diet, it is extremely important that you up your water intake as remaining in ketosis is naturally dehydrating. This means you are going to want to try and drink a gallon of water per day which means you are going to want to start carrying a water bottle with you wherever you go. As an added bonus, if you were previously drinking a large amount of soda then this should help you break that habit as well. Also, don't forget that if you are feeling thirsty then this means you are already dehydrated. Black coffee and tea are also viable options, providing you don't abuse them.

Alternatives to sugar: After you make it to ketosis it is still extremely important to monitor your sugar intake carefully to ensure it doesn't cause your insulin to spike to an unhealthy level. This transition is more than simply switching to a sugar substitute either as both maltodextrin and dextrose, common sugar substitutes, actively make it more difficult for you to remain in ketosis. Viable non-sugar sweeteners include stevia, erythritol, sucralose, xylitol, monk fruit, and agave nectar.

Spices: While most people rarely give the spices on their foods much thought, they can be a sneaky source of carbs if you aren't careful. While adding cayenne pepper to your food isn't going to add much to your overall daily carb intake, for example, when you only have a handful of grams to work with, every little bit counts. If you find that you just can't seem to remain in ketosis despite your best efforts then spices may very well be the culprit.

Fat bombs: With practically all of the carbs taken out of your diet, your body is likely to notice the difference, especially when it is craving something extra salty or extra sweet. Luckily, there is a keto-approved way to take care of these cravings which are known as the fat bomb. Fat bombs are an easy, quick and healthy snack that can be made to suit your tastes and is made up of at least 80 percent fat. Common fat bomb ingredients include things like seeds, butter, oil, coconut, and cheese, but the combinations are virtually endless.

While they are delicious, they are also nutritious which means that they will provide you will an instant burst of energy in a way that carb-based snacks will not. This makes them the perfect option when you are looking for a burst of energy for the gym or when you know you won't have time for a proper meal at the regular time. While they are certainly healthy, this doesn't mean that you are going to want to go crazy on them as they can still add up to more than you should eat in a day if you aren't careful. Generally speaking, try and stick with no more than two per day.

Chapter 3:
Keto Diet on the Go

While preparing something to eat at home that sticks to the keto diet is relatively straightforward, things become more complicated when you venture out into the wide world and are looking for something to eat that won't throw you out of ketosis. This chapter will cover the basics of what you should be able to count on regardless of what type of restaurant you find yourself at.

Italian: While the American version of Italian food doesn't stray too far beyond cheese and bread, you may be surprised to learn that a traditional Italian meal is comprised of far more than just these two ingredients. Pasta and pizza are very much staples in Italian food restaurants here in America and a big part of these dishes are the toppings, which usually consist of good meats and healthy veggies. Try ordering a pasta or pizza meal but ask for the toppings to go over lettuce. If you can, make sure the vegetables are cooked in olive oil, or even butter, if it's full fat. Grass fed is preferable but not always attainable. Choose straight olive oil and vinegar for the dressing, unless you've confirmed that their ranch or Caesar does not have excess amounts of sugar, especially if it's house-made.

Grilled chicken, beef, or fish will also most likely be on the menu, you'll just have to forgo carb-loaded sides and sauces. Pesto is an option to spread over chicken but use sparingly because of the pine nuts.

Antipasto ("before meal") platters are often available for appetizers. These plates usually consist of meats, vegetables, and sometimes seafood, all of which are excellent low-carb options.

Soups can be a good keto meal as well, as long as they are made with thinner broths rather than thicker "chowder" bases. Chowders often need starch and/or flour to make them thicken which will knock you out of ketosis very quickly. Steer clear of soups with pasta, beans, or gnocchi in them as well.

Mexican: Mexican cuisine is delicious and exciting, but much of it includes beans and rice in a variety of forms which is not conducive to staying in ketosis. Requesting meals without the rice and beans will immediately lower the carb count.

You can get just about any meal that comes in a tortilla either on the side or over a bed of shredded lettuce. Cheese, full fat sour cream, red salsas, and avocado are all keto approved. Watch out for the additives in guacamole. If you would rather have that over plain avocado slices, be sure to ask what the ingredients are. As a general rule if you are considering eating any meat that is grilled then you should be good to go with sides such as Pico de Gallo or ceviche spicing things up nicely.

Japanese: Much of Japanese cuisine, including many types of sushi are already low-carb which means you will be able to enjoy practically everything on the menu with little to no extra modification. Even still, you will want to go with sashimi instead of rice and to avoid edamame which contains 10 net carbs per serving.

Miso soup is a great keto-friendly starter that is surprisingly filling. Another great choice found at many Japanese restaurants is Konjac ramen which manages to remain low-carb despite being a noodle-based dish. This is because these noodles are actually made from the roots of the elephant yam and only contain about 3 net grams of carbs per serving. While there will be more in the bowl than just the noodles, they are certainly a viable item to build a healthy meal around.

As with most places, when you are unsure of what to order, grilled meat is always a viable choice, assuming you have a good idea what is in the sauce. Teriyaki bowls can always be ordered with the sauce on the side and can be a perfectly filling meal even if you leave the rice alone.

Indian: You may find that it is somewhat more difficult to find quality Indian cuisine that sticks to the keto diet. This doesn't mean it is impossible, however, it just means you are going to miss out on the spices and sauces that make this type of food stand out. Likewise, many of the dishes are full of extra sugars and flours as a means of thickening this or that.

As such, when ordering you are going to want to choose options that can have the sauce place on the side and you will obviously want to skip the rice and the naan. One common option that should be safe in most instances is the Tandoori chicken, as long as you get the marinade on the side. Kabobs are also a good choice because it is easy to avoid the items on the list that will push you out of ketosis.

Barbeque: When it comes to remaining in ketosis at a barbeque restaurant, the first thing you are going to want to look for is items that don't have any sauce whatsoever, which admittedly rather defeats the purpose of certain types of restaurants. You should still be able to find a dry-rub item that fits within the keto diet, sauce or no sauce. You will also want to stay away from dishes like barbacoa, pulled pork, or any other shredded meat as they are all generally prepared in sauce making them off limits. This all goes out the window if you can find a sauce made from mustard and vinegar which is perfectly keto friendly.

When it comes to wings, you should be alright with a dry-rub which is an option at popular chain Buffalo Wild Wings. You can typically also order them with the sauce on the side. Common sense salad and side rules apply in this scenario which means you are going to want to steer clear of sweets, dressing with fruit and anything breaded or fried.

Sports bars: The average sports bar these days should have a number of low-carb options on the menu. Unfortunately, if you are out with friends then it can be easy to lose track of things and find yourself eating whatever happens to be at the table. This is a dangerous mistake to make with ketosis on the line which means you need to be proactive and ensure you are making the order choices for the table or that you order your own items early to avoid having to deal with the temptation of eating poorly at the moment.

When in doubt, non-breaded chicken or steak are going to be found on most menus and there should be little the cook can do to hide extra carbs where you might not expect. Burgers, hold the bun, pork chops and grilled fish are all good choices as well. Just be mindful of the sides and you should be fine.

Really on the go

The following suggestions are for when you find yourself out and about with no time for a proper meal and little in the way of options. You should be able to find all of the following at your average bodega or gas station.

Cheese: While not without a few net carbs, a pack of string cheese can get some much needed fat into your system with no muss and no fuss. Just be sure that you are choosing a full-fat option and avoid eating more than one at a time.

Cold cuts: Most gas stations and bodegas have a refrigerated section that contains things like cold cuts. While not every option will be healthy, those that are not processed should be able to get you through. Wrap some salami around a serving of string cheese and you are 75 percent of the way to a fat bomb.

Beef jerky: While the extremely processed varieties are going to be full of unhealthy preservatives, those that are somewhat more stripped down can be a great source of protein, a reasonable source of fat and only a mild source of carbs. Ensure you stick with the unflavored versions, however, as the flavored options will contain far more carbs.

Pork rinds: While you might not think of pork rinds as being all that healthy, even the most processed version should contain a low enough amount of net carbs to make them a viable option in a pinch. While the flavor may take some getting used to, this is likely one of the best keto snacks you will find in many places with a limited selection.

Chapter 4:
Are You Doing the Keto Diet Correctly?

Entering ketosis: Once you have made the decision to adopt a ketogenic lifestyle, it is important to be aware of the fact that a state of ketosis will not be achieved after you skip a couple of low carb meals. Rather if you proceed down this path you will find that it will take as many as 7 days before you start to feel the effects of ketosis. Be warned, the interim period is likely going to be rough going as your body will be burning through all of its fuel reserves without having the benefit of ketones to pick up the slack. During this period, it is extremely important to stick to your guns as only cutting out carbohydrates slowly will only prolong your suffering.

Forewarned is forearmed, however, and there are a few things you can to in order to encourage your body to enter ketosis as quickly and easily as possible. First things first, if you are exercising regularly make sure you are doing so on an empty stomach as this will further reduce the leftover glucose in your body. Likewise, you may find that skipping an extra meal here or there will also get you to where you need to be more quickly. Essentially, any time your stomach is growling is a period of time that is actively pushing you towards a state of ketosis. Finally, during this period you are going to want to stick to a strict limit of 15 carbohydrates per day or less to get you to where you need to be.

Reading labels specifically for keto: Learning to read calories is not only important but absolutely vital, sure, and you'll want to pay attention to how many calories you consume. However, the best way to ease into keto is by simply becoming aware of carbs. Start reading labels of foods that you eat to look for their carbohydrates. This will also get you used to the idea of net carbs, which is central to keto. Net carbs are comprised of the carbs you eat which affect blood glucose. This means that the carbohydrates which don't affect blood glucose are unimportant. These may be listed as dietary fiber, sugar alcohols, or any other number of things.

If you aren't sure, run a Google search to learn whether or not the term affects blood glucose. To draw the net carbs, you just deduct the grams of dietary fiber and sugar alcohols from the total carbohydrates. The goal on Keto is to eat fewer than twenty grams of net carbs per day; other forms of carbohydrate don't matter, as they don't affect blood sugar, they are simply passed.

A big part of this will likely be eliminating your sweet tooth. If you travel abroad you will find that many other cultures find it bizarre how much sugar the Standard American Diet contains; indeed, once you wean yourself off of sugar, foods that you ate before start to seem too sweet by comparison.

Measure your ketones: So, where could you be going wrong with measuring your ketones? It could be a few different things. One, you could not be measuring at all and just expecting your body to do the work for you. Two, you could be measuring the wrong way or you not understand the concept of ketosis and how to stay in it.

One of the most accurate ways of measuring your ketones is with a blood ketone meter. The meter can determine the level of ketones in your blood and costs about $40 alone with the strips costing about $5 a piece. On the one hand, it is nice to have an accurate measurement, on the other, you could be using that extra money on food for your diet. If the number is vital to you, the blood ketone meter is most likely your best option.

Another good option for measuring your ketones is with urine ketone measuring strips. These strips are only able to show you the excess ketone bodies that you have excreted through your urine. This counts the number of acetoacetates. However, it does not tell you anything about the BHB in your bloodstream. In most cases, they are probably higher than the level the strip shows you. It should also be noted that these strips do not measure all of the types of ketones that your body produces.

Don't forget to exercise: In order to see some of the best results on this diet plan, you should add in a bit of exercise each day. This is going to help you to keep your heart happy and healthy and you will be able to burn up the fat inside the body faster than ever before. You should try to make a mix of different activities, combining together some stretching, weight lifting, and cardio.

In addition to making an effort to mix up the three main types of workouts that you are doing, you should also try out a few different types of activities in each group to ensure that you are working out different muscles and not getting bored with the work. For example, if the only thing that you do for your cardio is walking, you are going to find that after a few weeks you are completely bored of the process and won't want to do it any longer. Rather than just sticking with walking all the time, you should combine in a few different things, such as dancing, running, biking, swimming, and more. You should mix all of the categories of working out to ensure you get the results that you want.

Finding the tricks that you need to keep going with the ketogenic diet can be tough. You want to make sure that you are following this diet plan as closely as possible to ensure that you are staying in the state of ketosis, but it is sometimes easier said than done. With the help of some of these tips, you will be able to get started on the ketogenic diet and seeing the results that you want in no time.

Having a log of the food intake: When one is strictly on the keto diet, it becomes very easy to over consume carbs. This, therefore, means logging is a very fundamental part of the keto diet. It is the information age hence it is possible to download apps that will help with this. There are also websites that facilitate this. For the apps, there are those that are free and others you will have to pay for. Doesn't hurt to invest in your own health though. The process of logging will consequently assist an individual to comprehend their diet and find out which particular nutrients are deficient so they can take steps to correct this issue.

Listen to your body: It is very important to listen to one's body. Learn to do this. We are all unique and different which means our bodies respond differently to similar diets. It is possible that one may take some time to adjust to the keto diet. If after starting keto and giving it a full month for your body to adjust, if you still feel lousy then it is advisable that you adjust your diet accordingly. This may be either to have an increase in the quality carbs intake per day or by changing the diet the type of fat balance. This means it can be omega-3, omega-6, saturated or unsaturated. One may also consider switching their keto diet to one that is more sustainable.

Know the Terminology

As you begin your journey through the keto world, you will come across many terms or abbreviations that may seem foreign. This should help clarify some of the confusion:

- Artificial Sweetener (*AS*) provides a zero/reduced carb count.

- Bulletproof Coffee (*BPC*) is generally a mixture of coffee, oil, and butter. It is meant to give you a full feeling.

- *Fat Bomb*: To re-coop the day's fat content; this is usually packed with fats and a lot of oils. The Macaroon Keto Bomb is an example included in the *Snacks and Desserts* section.

- Heavy Whipping Cream (*HWC*) is used by many cooks.

- Insulin resistance (*IR*) (diabetes)

- Low-Carb and High-Fat (*LCHF*)

- Sugar-Free (*SF*)

- Way of Eating (*WOE*)

- Beta-hydroxybutyrate (BHB) is a ketone body found in the blood.

Chapter 5:
Worry-Free 14 Day Keto Diet Plan

Day 1

Breakfast: Celery Hash Browns

Total Prep & Cooking Time: 10 minutes
Yields: 6 Servings

Nutrition Stats (one serving)
- Protein: 5 grams
- Net Carbs: 0.2 grams
- Fats: 18.4 grams
- Calories: 185

What to Use
- Salt (1 pinch)
- Pepper (1 pinch
- Ghee (1 tsp.)
- Celery root (1)

What to Do
- Start by completely peeling the celery root before chopping it into manageable pieces for either processing with a food processor or grating by hand.
- Add the salt and pepper to the results as well as any other spices you would care to try.
- Place your frying pan on the stove on top of a high/medium heat before adding the 1 tsp. of ghee.
- Form the celery into the shape of hash browns in the frying pan, making them as small or as large as you would like. Smaller celery root hash browns will take less time to cook than larger versions and your cooking time should vary accordingly.
- Cook the celery root hash browns for around 15 minutes for an average sized hash brown.
- Flip the celery root has brown and brown the other side for about the same amount of time. It is important to not attempt to flip the hash brown until the first side is well-browned.

Lunch: Steak Salad

Total Prep & Cooking Time: 35 minutes
Yields: 4 Servings

Nutrition Stats (one serving)
- Protein: 25 grams
- Net Carbs: 5 grams
- Fats: 26 grams
- Calories: 451

What to Use
- Flat Iron Steak (1.5 lbs.)
- Fresh Garlic (2 cloves)
- Yellow Bell Pepper (1 medium)
- Orange Bell Pepper (1 medium)
- Chopped Romaine Lettuce (1 large head)
- Avocado (1 large)
- Sweet Onion (1 small)
- Cremini Mushrooms (about 3 or 4)
- Sundried Tomatoes (3oz can)
- Avocado Oil (3 T)
- Red Pepper Flakes (1 tsp.)
- Onion Powder (1 tsp.)
- Italian Seasoning (1 tsp.)
- Garlic Salt (1 tsp.)
- Balsamic Vinegar (0.25 c)
- Pink Himalayan Salt (0.25 tsp.)
- Ground Black Pepper (0.25 tsp.)

What to Do
- Cut steak into strips and place in large mixing bowl. Cover with balsamic vinegar then toss together until steak is completely dressed.
- Heat avocado oil over low-medium heat then add sliced mushrooms, sliced onion, garlic, salt, and pepper. Sauté vegetable mix until completely caramelized – usually 20 minutes.
- In the meantime, thinly slice bell peppers and chop romaine lettuce. Peel and pit your avocado and cut into wedges. Mix all fresh vegetables into bowl with sundried tomatoes.

- Grease broiling pan and line steak strips in a single layer, combine seasonings and sprinkle over steak. Broil on high on the top rack of your oven for 5 minutes for medium-rare or longer for more thoroughly cooked meat.
- Dish salad mixture on a plate and layer with the caramelized onion and mushrooms, then top with steak strips. Serve.

Dinner: Keto Meatloaf

Total Prep & Cooking Time: 85 minutes
Yields: 12 Servings

Nutrition Stats (one serving)
- Protein: 25 grams
- Net Carbs: 3.2 grams
- Fats: 33.6 grams
- Calories: 384

What to Use
- Almond flour (.5 c)
- Butter (2 T)
- Garlic (5 cloves Minced)
- Green pepper (1 c)
- Basil leaves (1 T)
- Thyme leaves (1 T)
- Parsley leaves (.25 c minced)
- Dijon mustard (2 tsp.)
- Barbeque sauce (2 T)
- Heavy cream (.25 c)
- Gelatin (.5 tsp. unflavored)
- Onion (8 oz. minced)
- Olive oil (1 T)
- Egg (2)
- Italian Sausage (1 lb.)
- Sea salt (1 tsp.)
- Pepper (. 5 tsp.)
- Parmesan cheese (.5 c)
- Ground beef (2 lb. lean)

What to Do
- Ensure that your oven has been preheated to 400F.

- Grease a 10X15 baking dish.
- This recipe requires a food processor.
- Combine the almond flour with the parmesan cheese.
- Coat a pan in olive oil and place it on the stove above a burner that has been turned to a medium heat.
- Add the peppers, onions, and garlic to the pan and let them sauté, you will be able to tell when they are finished because the onions will be practically see through.
- Let the pan cool before adding the ingredients to the food processor and processing well.
- Combine the gelatin, eggs, spices, salt, pepper, barbeque sauce, mustard, and cream. Let the mixture sit for at least 5 minutes before combining it with the processed garlic, peppers, and onion.
- Combine the sausage with the beef before adding all of the ingredients to a baking dish and shaping the results as desired.
- Place the dish in the oven and let it bake for roughly 60 minutes or until the center of meatloaf reaches 160F.
- Serve hot or cold and enjoy.

<u>Day 2</u>

Breakfast: Early Morning Meatballs

Total Prep & Cooking Time: 60 minutes
Yields: 6 Servings

Nutrition Stats (one serving)
- Protein: 19 grams
- Net Carbs: 4.9 grams
- Fats: 22.7 grams
- Calories: 269

What to Use
- Black pepper (as desired)
- Salt (as desired)
- Paprika (1 tsp.)
- Tomato sauce (.5 c)
- Eggs (2)
- Ground pork (2 lbs.)
- Bacon grease (1 T)
- Onion (1 c diced)

What to Do
- Cover a baking tray using parchment paper.
- Coat a skillet using the bacon grease before adding it to the stove above a burner turned to a medium/high heat.
- Place the onion in the skillet and let it cook for approximately 6 minutes until you can start to see through it.
- Let the onions cool before adding them and the ground pork to a large mixing bowl and combining thoroughly. Add in the eggs, tomato sauce, paprika, salt, and pepper before combining well and splitting the results into six equal portions.
- Place the results onto the covered baking tray, before adding the tray to the oven and letting it bake for approximately 45 minutes.
- Cut the meatballs in half, fill as desired, serve hot and enjoy.

Lunch: Cauliflower Bacon Bites

Total Prep & Cooking Time: 45 minutes
Yields: 10 Servings

Nutrition Stats (one serving)
- Protein: 12 grams
- Net Carbs: 2.2 grams
- Fats: 17.9 grams
- Calories: 190

What to Use
- Black pepper (as desired)
- Salt (as desired)
- Garlic Powder (1 tsp.)
- Onion powder (1 tsp.)
- Italian seasoning (1 tsp. divided)
- Garlic (3 cloves minced)
- Panko (.5 c)
- Crushed pork rinds (1 c)
- White cheddar cheese (.5 c)
- Sharp cheddar cheese (.5 c)
- Parmesan cheese (1.5 c divided)
- Goat cheese (4 oz.)
- Cream cheese (8 oz. softened)
- Bacon (1 lb. crumbled, cooked)
- Cauliflower rice (5 c)

What to Do
- Turn the cauliflower into rice by processing it using a food processor.
- Mix together the salt, pepper, .5 tsp. Italian seasoning, minced garlic, .5 c grated parmesan cheese, white cheddar cheese, sharp cheddar cheese, goat cheese, cream cheese, bacon and cauliflower in a mixing bowl. Place the bowl in the refrigerator for 60 minutes.
- In a separate bowl, combine the Italian seasoning, garlic powder, onion powder, panko, parmesan cheese, and pork rinds and mix well.
- Once it has cooled, roll the contents of the first bowl into balls before coating with the mixture in the second bowl.

- About roughly 1 inch of oil to a large frying pan before placing it on the stove above a burner turned to a high/ medium heat. Once the oil heats up, add in 5 of the balls at a time and fry for 6 minutes so they are golden brown.

Dinner: Cinnamon and Orange Beef Stew

Total Prep & Cooking Time: 10 minutes
Yields: 6 Servings

Nutrition Stats (one serving)
- Protein: 43.5 grams
- Net Carbs: 1.9 grams
- Fats: 44.5 grams
- Calories: 649

What to Use
- Bay leaf (1)
- Sage (.25 tsp.)
- Rosemary (.25 tsp.)
- Fish sauce (.5 tsp.)
- Soy sauce (.5 tsp.)
- Cinnamon (.5 tsp. ground)
- Garlic (.75 tsp. minced)
- Thyme (.75 tsp.)
- Orange (.25 juiced)
- Orange (.25 zest)
- Onion (.25 medium)
- Coconut oil (1 T)
- Beef broth (.75 c)
- Beef (.5 lbs. cubed)

What to Do
- This recipe can easily be doubled or tripled if you want to set aside extra for leftovers.
- You are going to want to start by adding the coconut oil to your skillet before setting over a burned turned to a high heat and letting it reach the smoke point.
- Add in the meat in batches and season as desired. Let each batch of beef brown completely prior to moving on to the next batch of beef.
- After all of the beef has browned, add in the onion and garlic and let them cook for 1.5 minutes before adding in the

orange juice, bay, fish sauce, orange zest, soy sauce, cinnamon, and thyme.
- Let the results cook for 20 seconds before adding it all to the slow cooker along with the remaining seasonings.
- Cover your slow cooker and let it cook on a high heat for 1.5 hours.

Day 3

Breakfast: Breakfast Ketogenic Eggs

Total Prep & Cooking Time: 20 minutes
Yields: 4 Servings

Nutrition Stats (one serving)
- Protein: 73 grams
- Net Carbs: 2.3 grams
- Fats: 15 grams
- Calories: 172

What to Use
- Shallot (1 T chopped)
- Ghee (3 T)
- Jalapeno (1 sliced)
- Cinnamon (1 tsp. ground)
- Cumin seeds (1 tsp. ground)
- Garlic (3 sliced cloves)
- Turmeric (.5 tsp.)
- Ginger (.5 tsp. ground)
- Salt (.5 tsp.)
- Eggs (4 beaten)

What to Do
- Add the ghee to the Instant Pot. Melt using the sauté function and add the cumin seeds, cooking until aromatic.
- Continue cooking for 3 minutes along with the shallots. Stir in the garlic. Sauté 3 additional minutes and add the salt, ginger, salt, and turmeric.
- Whisk in the eggs and cook until set (30 sec.). When the eggs are at the right texture, sprinkle with the pepper, salt, and cilantro.
- Secure the lid and prepare for 13 minutes. Quick release the steam and serve.

Lunch: Chicken with Roasted Vegetables

Total Prep & Cooking Time: 30 minutes
Yields: 4 Servings

Nutrition Stats (one serving)
- Protein: 28 grams
- Net Carbs: 6.8 grams
- Fats: 27 grams
- Calories: 401

What to Use
- Salt (as desired)
- Pepper (as desired)
- Coconut oil (2 T)
- Oregano (.5 T dried)
- Rosemary (1.5 T)
- Garlic (2 cloves smashed)
- Balsamic vinegar (.25 c + 1 T)
- Mushrooms (5 oz. sliced)
- Red bell peppers (2 sliced)
- Asparagus (10 spears cut in half)
- Chicken thighs (8, 4 oz. apiece)

What to Do
- Start by making sure your oven is heated to 425F.
- Mix the salt and pepper together in a small bowl before using the results to coat the chicken thoroughly.
- Prepare two baking sheets by spraying them with cooking spray.
- Add all of the ingredients to a large mixing bowl and mix well. Spread the results so they form an even layer across both baking sheets. Ensure that none of the vegetables are touching the chicken so they roast rather than steam.
- Place the baking sheets in the oven for about 20 minutes or until the chicken reaches at least 165F and the vegetables are tender.

Dinner: Steak Seared in Port Sauce

Total Prep & Cooking Time: 20 minutes
Yields: 4 Servings

Nutrition Stats (one serving)
- Protein: 41 grams
- Net Carbs: 5.2 grams
- Fats: 38.4 grams
- Calories: 485

What to Use
- Strip steak (1.25 lbs.)
- Kosher salt (.5 tsp.)
- Pepper (.25 tsp.)
- Coconut oil (1 T)
- Seedless red grapes (1 c)
- Shallot (.25 c diced)
- Wheat flour (1.5 tsp.)
- Port wine (.25 c)
- Beef bone broth (.25 c)
- Thyme (1 tsp. chopped)

What to Do
- Start by quartering the steak and seasoning as desired.
- Add the coconut oil to a pan before adding the pan to the stove over a low/medium heat.
- Let the steak cooked as preferred.
- Remove the steak from the pan and cover it with tinfoil to ensure it remains warm.
- Place the grapes in the pan and let them cook for 4 minutes, stirring and pressing on them regularly.
- Add in the shallot and let it cook until it begins to become fragrant.
- Add in the flour and ensure everything is well coated.
- Add in the salt, broth, thyme, and port before turning the temperature to high/medium and letting everything cook for an additional 2 minutes.
- Add the sauce to the steak, serve hot and enjoy.

Day 4

Breakfast: Shakshuka

Total Prep & Cooking Time: 45 minutes
Yields: 4 Servings

Nutrition Stats (one serving)
- Protein: 26.1 grams
- Net Carbs: 4.5 grams
- Fats: 41.6 grams
- Calories: 571

What to Use
- Eggs (5)
- Pepper (as desired)
- Salt (as desired)
- Chili powder (.25 tsp.)
- Paprika (1 tsp.)
- Cumin powder (1 tsp.)
- Tomatoes (1.5 chopped)
- Bell pepper (.5 chopped)
- Serrano pepper (.25 chopped)
- Garlic (1.5 cloves chopped)
- White onion (.5 chopped)
- Ghee (2 T)

What to Do
- Add the ghee to a skillet before placing it on the stove over a medium heat and adding in the onion. Let it cook for approximately 10 minutes, stirring consistently until it begins to soften.
- Add in the serrano pepper along with the garlic and let them cook for 2 minutes before adding in the red bell pepper and turning the heat to low. Let all the ingredients cook an additional 10 minutes, stirring consistently.
- Mix in the tomatoes and the remaining spices before letting the dish simmer and continue cooking until the sauce has reduced to your desired level.

- Add the eggs to the skillet before seasoning as desired and letting everything cook, covered for approximately 5 minutes until the eggs reach your desired level of doneness.

Lunch: Meat Pie

Total Prep & Cooking Time: 70 minutes
Yields: 6 Servings

Nutrition Stats (one serving)
- Protein: 28.1 grams
- Net Carbs: 4.4 grams
- Fats: 33.6 grams
- Calories: 415

What to Use - Filling
- Water (.5 c)
- Tomato paste (4 T)
- Dried oregano (1 T)
- Sea salt (as desired)
- Black pepper (as desired)
- Ground lamb (1.3 lbs.)
- Olive oil (2 T)
- Garlic (1 clove chopped fine)
- Yellow onion (.5 chopped fine)

What to Use - Crust
- Water (4 T)
- Egg (1 large, organic)
- Coconut oil (3 T)
- Salt (1 pinch)
- Baking powder (1 tsp.)
- Psyllium husk powder (1 T)
- Coconut powder (4 T)
- Sesame seeds (4 T)
- Almond flour (.75 c)

What to Use - Toppings
- Shredded cheese (7 oz.)
- Cottage cheese (8 oz.)

What to Do

- Ensure your oven is heated to 350F.
- Add the olive oil to a skillet before placing it on the stove over a burned turned to a high/medium heat. Add in the garlic along with the onion and let them fry for 3 minutes or until they have softened.
- Add in the ground beef, basil and oregano and season as desired before adding in the tomato paste as well as the water. Reduce the heat and let everything simmer 20 minutes. While this is taking place, make the crust.
- Combine the dough ingredients using a food processor and process until the results form a ball. The same effect can be achieved by hand mixing with a fork.
- Line greased 10-inch springform pan before spreading in the dough.
- Bake the crust for 15 minutes before removing it and adding in the filling.
- Mix together the shredded cheese and cottage cheese and add this on top.
- Bake 30 minutes and let sit 5 minutes prior to baking.

Dinner: Bacon Chicken Chowder

Total Prep & Cooking Time: 10 minutes
Yields: 6 Servings

Nutrition Stats (one serving)

- Protein: 21 grams
- Net Carbs: 3.4 grams
- Fats: 28 grams
- Calories: 355

What to Do

- Salt (as desired)
- Pepper (as desired)
- Thyme (1 tsp. dried)
- Garlic powder (1 tsp.)
- Bacon (1 lb. well-cooked, crumbled)
- Heavy cream (1 c)
- Cream cheese (8 oz.)
- Chicken breast (1 lb.)

- Chicken stock (2 c divided)
- Butter (4 T divided)
- Sweet onion (1 sliced thin)
- Mushrooms (6 oz. sliced)
- Celery (2 ribs diced)
- Leek (1 sliced, trimmed, cleaned)
- Shallot (1 chopped fine)
- Garlic (4 cloves minced)

What to Use
- Turn the slow cooker to low before adding in the pepper, salt, 1 c of the chicken stock, 2 T butter, onions, mushrooms, celery, leek, shallot, and garlic. Cover the slow cooker and let the vegetables cook for 60 minutes.
- While the vegetables cook, place a large skillet on top of the stove over a burner turned to a medium/high heat. Add in the chicken along with the rest of the butter and let it cook until both sides are browned or approximately 5 minutes per side.
- Remove the chicken from the pan and use the rest of the chicken stock for the deglazing process. Scrape up any remaining chicken pieces and then add everything in the pan to the slow cooker.
- Add in the thyme, garlic powder, cream cheese, and heavy cream and mix well to combine.
- Cube the chicken and add the results to the slow cooker before mixing in the bacon and combining thoroughly.
- Adjust the slow cooker temperature to low and leave it be, covered, for at least 6 hours or until the chicken's internal temp has met or exceeded 165 degrees.

Day 5

Breakfast: Macadamia Nut Smoothie

Total Prep & Cooking Time: 5 minutes
Yields: 1 Servings

Nutrition Stats (one serving)
- Protein: 7.2 grams
- Net Carbs: 6.4 grams
- Fats: 44.7 grams
- Calories: 412

What to Use
- Ice cubes (6)
- Your choice of sweetener (as desired)
- Coconut milk (.75 c)
- Macadamia nuts (3 T)
- Cocoa (1 T)
- Salt (1 dash)
- Toasted coconut (1 t)

What to Do
- Cream the coconut milk: This is a simple process. All you need to do is place the can of coconut milk in the refrigerator overnight. The next morning, open the can and spoon out the coconut milk that has solidified. Don't shake the can before opening. Discard the liquids.
- Add all of the ingredients, save the ice cubes, to the blender and blend on a low speed until pureed. Thin with water as needed.
- Add in the ice cubes and blend until the smoothie reaches your desired consistency.

Lunch: Ketogenic Tuna Melt

Total Prep & Cooking Time: 20 minutes
Yields: 1 Serving

Nutrition Stats (one serving)
- Protein: 25 grams

- Net Carbs: 3.1 grams
- Fats: 29.7 grams
- Calories: 444

What to Use - Bread
- Powdered psyllium husk (.5 T)
- Salt (.25 tsp)
- Eggs (3)
- Cream cheese (4 oz)

What to Use - Filling
- Salt (as desired)
- Pepper (as desired)
- Shredded cheddar cheese (4 oz)
- Lemon juice (.5 tsp)
- Garlic cloves (.5 minced)
- Olive oil (1 can)
- Sour cream (.3 c)
- Dill pickles (.25 c chopped)
- Celery stalk (1)

What to Do - Bread
- Ensure your oven is on and turned to 300F.
- Break the eggs and separate the whites from the yolks in different bowls.
- Mix together the whites with the salt and whisk vigorously.
- Mix together the yolks with the cream cheese and then add in the powdered psyllium and the baking powder.
- Combine the contents of both bowls and mix well before adding the mixture to a baking sheet and forming it into 8 slices
- Place the baking sheet in the center of the oven and bake for 25 minutes.

What to Do -Filling
- Turn the oven to 350F.
- In a mixing bowl, add all of the filling ingredients except for the shredded cheese and mix thoroughly.
- Line a baking sheet before placing 2 of the bread slices onto it and topping them with the filling. Add the cheese last.

- Place the baking sheet in the oven and let it bake for 15 minutes.

Dinner: Grilled Pork Chops

Total Prep & Cooking Time: 55 minutes
Yields: 6 Servings

Nutrition Stats (one serving)
- Protein: 31 grams
- Net Carbs: 1.2 grams
- Fats: 36.9 grams
- Calories: 532

What to Use
- Scallions (6)
- Salt (.5 tsp.)
- Pepper (as desired)
- Avocados (2 mashed)
- Green beans (.75 lbs.)
- Olive oil (2 T)
- Pork shoulder chops (4)
- Olive Oil (2 T)
- Chipotle paste (2 T)
- Onion (.5 chopped)

What to Do
- Start by making sure your oven is heated to 400F.
- In a small mixing bowl combine the chipotle, salt and oil and mix well.
- Add the results to the pork and let it sit for 15 minutes to marinate.
- Place the pork on a baking sheet and let it bake for 30 minutes, turning after 15 minutes.
- While the pork cooks add the oil to a frying pan before placing it on the stove over a burner set to a medium heat before adding in the beans and letting them cook 5 minutes. For the last minute turn the heat to low and season as desired.
- Add the onion and the avocado into the beans to warm and season as needed prior to plating with the pork chops.

Day 6

Breakfast: Crepes with Cream and Raspberries

Total Prep & Cooking Time: 10 minutes
Yields: 6 Servings

Nutrition Stats (one serving)
- Protein: 15 grams
- Net Carbs: 6 grams
- Fats: 40 grams
- Calories: 226

What to Use
- Raspberries (3 oz., fresh or frozen)
- Whole Milk Ricotta (.5 c + 2 T)
- Erythritol (2 T)
- Eggs (2 large)
- Cream Cheese (2 oz.)
- Salt (1 pinch)
- Cinnamon (1 dash)

What to Do
- In a blender, blend cream cheese, eggs, erythritol, salt, and cinnamon for about 20 seconds, or until there are no lumps of cream cheese.
- Place a pan on a burner turned to a medium heat before coating in cooking spray. Add 20 percent of your batter to the pan in a thin layer. Cook crepe until the underside becomes slightly darkened. Carefully flip the crepe and let the reverse side cook for about 15 seconds.
- Repeat step 3 until all batter is used.
- Without stacking the crepes, allow them to cool for a few minutes.
- After the crepes have cool, place about 2 T of ricotta cheese in the center of each crepe.
- Throw in a couple of raspberries and fold the side to the middle.

Lunch: Chicken Soup

Total Prep & Cooking Time: 35 minutes
Yields: 1 Serving

Nutrition Stats (one serving)
- Protein: 15 grams
- Net Carbs: 4.2 grams
- Fats: 32 grams
- Calories: 280

What to Use
- Salt (as desired)
- Pepper (as desired)
- Chicken (6 oz. shredded)
- Celery stalks (3)
- Olive oil (40 ml)
- Cayenne (.5 tsp powdered)
- Bell pepper (1, red)
- Garlic (1 tsp., minced)
- Chicken broth (200 ml)
- Tomatoes (1 c, diced)
- Cream cheese (6 oz.)
- Cilantro (2 oz.)
- Cumin (1 tsp)

What to Do
- Dice the celery and the bell pepper.
- Add the olive oil to a skillet before placing the skillet on top of a burner set to a medium heat.
- Add in celery, bell pepper, and the garlic until the celery softens.
- Season as desired.
- Mix in tomatoes. Stir constantly.
- Mix in the broth along with the chicken and let everything cook approximately 4 minutes.
- Mix in remaining spices.
- Stir well. Let everything cook 2 additional minutes
- Mix in the chopped cilantro.
- Boil and turn the burner to low.
- Mix in cream cheese until it melts in.

- Boil for another 5 minutes.
- Put into serving bowls and garnish with diced tomatoes and cilantro leaves.

Dinner: Sticky Sweet Honey Teriyaki Chicken

Total Prep & Cooking Time: 30 minutes
Yields: 8 Servings

Nutrition Stats (one serving)
- Protein: 15.7 grams
- Net Carbs: 2.7 grams
- Fats: 42 grams
- Calories: 203

What to Use
- Rice vinegar (.3 c)
- Chicken breast (4 skinless, boneless)
- Low-sodium soy sauce (.5 c)
- Onion (.5 sliced)
- Ginger (.6 tsp. ground)
- Garlic cloves (2 crushed)
- Pepper (.25 tsp.)
- Organic honey (.5 c)
- Cornstarch (3 T)
- Sesame seeds (as desired)
- Water (.3 c)
- Onion (.3 c sliced)

What to Do
- Use non-stick cooking spray to spray the inside of the Instant Pot inner pot
- Place chicken breasts into the inner pot
- Whisk together honey, soy sauce, rice vinegar, crushed garlic, onion, and seasonings together and use the results to coat the chicken.
- Cook for 17 minutes on high pressure. Check to see if the chicken is cooked. Once cooled slightly, remove from Instant pot and shred chicken.
- Combine the water and cornstarch. Slowly incorporate the sauce inside the Instant Pot and press 'Sauté' while whisking

the mixture. Allow the pan to sauté for a minute till the sauce begins to boil and thicken.

- Turn off the pot and place shredded chicken into the pot and stir with the sauce to coat.
- Serve chicken over rice and garnish with sesame seeds and green onions.

Day 7

Breakfast: Egg Bake

Total Prep & Cooking Time: 30 minutes
Yields: 4 Servings

Nutrition Stats (one serving)
- Protein: 15 grams
- Net Carbs: 2.2 grams
- Fats: 23.8 grams
- Calories: 280

What to Use
- Pepper (as desired)
- Red pepper flakes (.25 tsp.)
- Parmesan cheese (.5 c grated)
- Eggs (4 large)
- Basil (.25 c chopped)
- Marinara sauce (2 c)

What to Do
- Start by making sure your oven is heated to 350F and your oven rack is in the middle of the oven.
- Add the marinara to a baking dish and coat the bottom well before adding in the basil. Form 4 furrows in the marinara and add an egg to each. Top the eggs with the red pepper flakes and parmesan cheese.
- Place the baking dish in the oven for approximately 19 minutes until the egg whites have set and the yolk is firm.
- Split the sauce amongst the serving bowls and add an egg to each.

Lunch: Cheesy Chicken

Total Prep & Cooking Time: 40 minutes
Yields: 2 Servings

Nutrition Stats (one serving)
- Protein: 30.7 grams
- Net Carbs: 5.4 grams
- Fats: 18.3 grams
- Calories: 330

What to Use
- Black pepper (as desired)
- Cream cheese (2 oz.)
- Cheddar cheese (2 oz.)
- Chicken breast (1 lb.)
- Bacon (2 slices)
- Water (1 c)
- Ranch seasoning (1 packet)
- Cornstarch (1.5 T)

What to Do
- Turn the instant pot cooker to sauté before adding in the bacon and allowing it to cook until it is crisp enough to crumble.
- Place the chicken in the instant pot cooker before topping it with the cream cheese and seasoning as desired.
- Add 1 c water to the pot and seal the lid of the cooker. Choose the high-pressure option and set the time for 25 minutes.
- Once the timer goes off, select the instant pressure release option and remove the lid before removing the chicken and shredding it with a pair of forks.
- Turn the heat on the instant pot cooker to low before adding in the cornstarch and whisking well. Add in the cheese and then return the chicken to the pot along with the bacon and mix well.
- Serve hot.

Dinner: Beef Lasagna

Total Prep & Cooking Time: 8 hours and 10 minutes
Yields: 10 Servings

Nutrition Stats (one serving)
- Protein: 29 grams
- Net Carbs: 3 grams
- Fats: 29 grams
- Calories: 224

What to Use
- Parmesan cheese (.5 c shredded)
- Lasagna Zoodles (6)
- Mozzarella cheese (1.5 c shredded)
- Ricotta cheese (1 c)
- Red pepper flakes (.25 tsp.)
- Basil (.5 tsp. dried)
- Oregano (1 tsp. dried)
- Salt (1 tsp.)
- Tomato sauce (15 oz.)
- Tomato (28 oz. crushed)
- Garlic (1 clove minced)
- Onion (1 chopped)
- Ground beef (1 lb.)

What to Do
- Place a skillet on the stove on top of a burner set to a high/ medium heat before adding in the garlic, onion, and beef and letting the beef brown.
- Add in the red pepper flakes, basil, oregano, salt, tomato sauce, and crushed tomatoes and let the results simmer 5 minutes.
- Combine the mozzarella and the ricotta cheese.
- Add .3 of the total sauce from the skillet and add it to the slow cooker. Place 3 Zoodles on top of the sauce, followed by cheese mixture. Create three layers total.
- Cover the slow cooker and let it cook on a low heat for 6 hours.

Day 8

Breakfast: Eggs Benedict

Total Prep & Cooking Time: 15 minutes
Yields: 4 Servings

Nutrition Stats (one serving)
- Protein: 5 grams
- Net Carbs: 5.1 grams
- Fats: 22.4 grams
- Calories: 177

What to Use
- Black pepper (as desired)
- Sea salt (as desired)
- Grass-fed butter (4 tsp.)
- Lemon juice (.5 T)
- Dijon mustard (.5 T)
- Light mayonnaise (1 T)
- Full-fat Greek Yogurt (.3)
- Apple cider vinegar (1 T)
- Eggs (4)
- Olive oil (1 tsp.)
- Tomato (4 slices)
- Canadian bacon (4 slices)
- Flatbread (4 slices)

What to Do
- Add enough water to a skillet to fill it halfway full before adding in the vinegar and placing it on the stove over a burner turned to a high heat. All the mixture to boil before turning down the heat and allowing the skillet to simmer. Add the eggs in one at a time and allow them to cook about 4 minutes.
- Separately, add 1 tsp olive oil to another pan before placing it on a burner turned to a high/medium heat. Add the bacon and allow it to cook until it reaches your desired level of crispiness.

- In a bowl that is microwave safe, combine the lemon juice, mustard, mayo, and yogurt and whisk well. Place the bowl in the microwave for 30 seconds before stirring in the butter.
- Top the flatbread with the egg, tomato, bacon, sauce, and seasoning prior to serving.

Lunch: Vegan Bibimbap

Total Prep & Cooking Time: 10 minutes
Yields: 6 Servings

Nutrition Stats (one serving)
- Protein: 8 grams
- Net Carbs: 0 grams
- Fats: 18 grams
- Calories: 119

What to Use
- Cucumber (.5 sliced into strips)
- Carrot (1 grated)
- Red bell pepper (1 sliced)
- Soy sauce (1 T)
- Sesame oil (1 tsp.)
- Cauliflower (10 oz. riced)
- Rice vinegar (2 T)
- Sesame seeds (2 T)
- Sriracha sauce (2 T)
- Broccoli florets (4)
- Tempeh (7 oz. sliced into squares)
- Liquid sweetener (as desired)

What to Do
- In a bowl, combine tempeh squares with 1 T soy sauce and 2 T vinegar. Set aside to soak. Slice veggies.
- Add carrot, broccoli, and peppers to slow cooker. Cook on high 30 minutes.
- Add cauliflower rice to the pot, cook 5 minutes.
- Add sweetener, oil, soy sauce, vinegar, and sriracha to slow cooker. Don't hesitate to add a bit of water if you find the mixture to be too thick.

Dinner: Spicy Cauliflower with Shirataki Noodles

Total Prep & Cooking Time: 20 minutes
Yields: 4 Servings

Nutrition Stats (one serving)
- Protein: 5.8 grams
- Net Carbs: 6.7 grams
- Fats: 12.8 grams
- Calories: 324

What to Use - Sauce
- Arrowroot powder (3 tsp.)
- Water (.25 c)
- Unrefined sugar (2 T)
- Gluten free soy sauce (4 T)
- Ketchup (2 T)
- Rice wine vinegar (2 T)

What to Use - Meal
- Shirataki noodles (1 lb.)
- Olive oil (2 T)
- Red pepper flakes (1 tsp.)
- Cashews (.3 c raw)
- Scallion (5 cut in 2 inch pieces)
- Garlic (2 cloves minced)
- Ginger (1 T minced)
- Orange pepper (1 diced)
- Yellow pepper (1 diced)
- Red pepper (1 diced)
- Cauliflower head (1 large, cut into florets)

What to Do
- Start by cooking the noodles as per the directions on the packaging.
- In a small bowl, combine the arrowroot powder, .25 c water, unrefined sugar, soy sauce, ketchup, and rice wine vinegar together and mix well.
- Place your skillet on the stove over a burner set to a medium heat before adding in the olive oil. Mix in the cauliflower and

let it cook for 5 minutes, stirring as needed before removing it from the skillet.

- Add in the orange pepper, yellow pepper, and red pepper and let them cook for 3 minutes before adding the cauliflower back in and letting everything cook for 5 minutes more.
- Mix in the cashews, ginger, and garlic and let them cook for 2 minutes before adding in the sauce, turning the heat on the skillet up to high and letting it cook for 1 minute until it thickens.
- Mix in the spring onions before serving on top of the noodles.

Day 9

Breakfast: Sausage Pie

Total Prep & Cooking Time: 40 minutes
Yields: 4 Servings

Nutrition Stats (one serving)
- Protein: 17 grams
- Net Carbs: 3 grams
- Fats: 32 grams
- Calories: 350

What to Use
- Bacon/chicken sausages (2)
- Cheddar cheese (.75 c grated)
- Coconut flour (.25 c)
- Coconut oil (.25 c)
- Coconut milk (2 T)
- Eggs (5 yolk only)
- Lemon juice (2 tsp.)
- Rosemary (.25 tsp.)
- Cayenne pepper (.25 tsp.)
- Baking soda (.25 tsp.)
- Kosher salt (1 dash)

What to Do
- Preheat your oven to 350F

- Take your bacon and chicken sausage and cut it into small cubes. Add the cubes to a pan and cook until slightly brown. (Depending on the brand of sausage you may or may not need to add oil. Fattier sausage will cook just fine without any extra oil.) Set the sausages when done cooking.
- Take a medium size mixing bowl and add your rosemary, cayenne, baking soda, salt, and coconut flour.
- Take a small bowl and add your egg yolks. Whisk until creamy and then add your coconut oil, coconut milk, and lemon juice. Continue to whisk the egg yolks and wet ingredients until it is well mixed.
- Take the small mixing bowl of wet ingredients and slowly mix it into the dry bowl. Make sure you do this very slowly as dumping it all in will make it very difficult to make the batter the right consistency.
- Place the batter into the 2 ramekins. You will want to use all of the batter but leave enough room so that you can add the cooked sausage on top.
- Place the sausage in the batter, pushing it through the batter to reach spots all throughout each ramekin.
- Bake for 22-25 minutes, topping each pie with shredded cheddar when they are fully cooked.
- Wait 3 minutes to cool and serve.

Lunch: Ham and Cheese Stromboli

Total Prep & Cooking Time: 30 minutes
Yields: 1 Serving

Nutrition Stats (one serving)
- Protein: 25.6 grams
- Net Carbs: 4 grams
- Fats: 21.8 grams
- Calories: 305

What to Use
- Egg (1 large)
- Mozzarella cheese (1.25 c shredded)
- Coconut flour (3 T)
- Almond flour (4 T)
- Ham (4 oz.)

- Italian seasoning (1 tsp.)
- Cheddar cheese (3.5 oz.)

What to Do
- Preset the oven to 400F oven.
- Melt the mozzarella cheese in the microwave for 1 minute/ alternating at 10-second intervals—stirring until entirely melted.
- In a mixing container, blend the coconut and almond flour with the seasonings.
- Add the mozzarella on the top and work it in.
- After the cheese has cooled; add the egg and combine everything
- On a flat surface; place some parchment paper and add the mixture.
- Use your hand or a rolling pin to flatten the mix.
- Place several diagonal lines using a knife or pizza cutter. (Leave a row of approximately four inches wide in the center.
- Alternate the cheddar and ham on the uncut space of dough until you have used all of the filling.
- Bake for 15 to 20 minutes or it is browned.

Dinner: Cheeseburger Muffins

Total Prep & Cooking Time: 40 minutes
Yields: 6 Servings

Nutrition Stats (one serving)
- Protein: 15 grams
- Net Carbs: 3 grams
- Fats: 19 grams
- Calories: 250

What to Use - Meat
- Ground beef (15 oz.)
- Garlic and onion powder (.5 tsp)
- Tomato paste (2 T)

What to Use – Buns
- Eggs (2)
- Flaxseed meal (.5 c)

- Almond flour (1 c)
- Sour cream (.5 c)

What to Use - Toppings
- Mustard (1 T)
- Ketchup (1 T)
- Cheddar cheese (.5 c shredded)
- Dill pickles (as desired)

What to Do
- First, you will want to cook your beef once you have seasoned with salt and pepper.
- In another bowl, mix all of your dry ingredients from above. This will be the makings of your bun. As you combine these, preheat your oven to 350 degrees.
- Once the dry ingredients for buns are put together, throw in the eggs and sour cream.
- As you fill the muffin wells, create indents in the muffins, so you have space to fill with meat.
- When the beef is placed, go ahead and bake for 15-20 minutes.
- Once the beef and muffins turn a golden brown, add some cheese on top and cook for another 5 minutes.
- Top with condiments and pickles as desired

Day 10

Breakfast: Asparagus and Cheese Frittata

Total Prep & Cooking Time: 50 minutes
Yields: 4 Servings

Nutrition Stats (one serving)
- Protein: 21.1 grams
- Net Carbs: 4.6 grams
- Fats: 34.7 grams
- Calories: 212

What to Use
- Dry white wine (.5 c.)
- Onion (.5)
- Thyme (.5 tsp. dried)
- Salt (.5 tsp.)
- Heavy cream (.25 c.)
- Butter (4 T)
- Swiss cheese (1 c. shredded)
- Cooking spray (2 T)
- Parmesan cheese (.5 c)
- Asparagus (1 lb.)
- Eggs (8)

What to Do
- Take out the asparagus and chop each of the stalks into small pieces. Grease up a skillet well with some of the cooking spray and then place on a medium heat.
- Add the onion and butter cook inside a skillet until soft. Add in the asparagus at this time and cook for a few minutes.
- Place all of the ingredients together in a container before pouring into the skillet. Stir it around until the asparagus and onions are distributed well.
- Adjust the heat to a low setting and cover the skillet. Cook this for about 20 minutes. At this time, check the frittata; if it is still runny, cook for another 5 minutes.
- When the frittata is almost done, move it over to the oven and broil for about 6 minutes before serving.

Lunch: Salmon Pizza

Total Prep & Cooking Time: 40 minutes
Yields: 3 Servings

Nutrition Stats (one serving)
- Protein: 31 grams
- Net Carbs: 6.2 grams
- Fats: 29.7 grams
- Calories: 420

What to Use
- Egg (1 large)
- Cream cheese (3 T)
- Cauliflower (1 head)
- Salmon (.5 c. cooked)
- Cheese (1 c)
- Tomato sauce (3 T)
- Olive oil (2 T)

What to Do
- Boil some water in a pan. Add the chopped up cauliflower and cook for 7 minutes. While cooking, turn on the oven to 350F.
- When the cauliflower is done, put into a bowl with the cream cheese, egg, oil, and seasoning and mix together.
- Spread this out onto a baking sheet and make into a crust. Throw into the and let this cook for 12 minutes.
- Remove at this time and add in the tomato sauce, cheese, and salmon. Put back into the oven.
- Bake for another 8 minutes so everything is melted and warm.

Dinner: Garlic Lemon Shrimp Pasta

Total Prep & Cooking Time: 20 minutes
Yields: 4 Servings

Nutrition Stats (one serving)
- Protein: 36 grams
- Net Carbs: 4 grams
- Fats: 21 grams
- Calories: 360

What to Use
- Ghee (2 T)
- Olive Oil (2 T)
- Paprika (0.5 tsp.)
- Shirataki Noodles (2 bags)
- Large, Raw Shrimp (1 lb.)
- Garlic Cloves (4)
- Lemon (.5)
- Salt (1 pinch)
- Pepper (1 pinch)
- Basil (1 pinch)

What to Do
- Begin by cooking noodles according to package directions.
- When done, transfer noodles to medium saucepan and heat over medium temperature. Cook until noodles are dry and roasted. Take the noodles off of the stove.
- Add in the fresh ghee along with the oil and heat until melted, then add crushed garlic cloves and cook until fragrant. Don't brown the garlic.
- Slice half of a lemon into thin slices and add to pan, then add shrimp. Let shrimp cook for 3 minutes on either side. Add noodles, paprika, salt, and pepper.
- Stir together and continue cooking until ingredients are well blended and noodles are thoroughly coated with flavoring. Remove from heat and serve.

Day 11

Breakfast: Keto Porridge

Total Prep & Cooking Time: 10 minutes
Yields: 1 Serving

Nutrition Stats (one serving)
- Protein: 12.3 grams
- Net Carbs: 5.1 grams
- Fats: 17.6 grams
- Calories: 201

What to Use
- Flaxseed (1 T)
- Cinnamon (1 tsp)
- Chia seeds (1 T)
- Sea salt (.25 tsp)
- Unsweetened coconut (2 T)
- Walnuts (.25 c)
- Water (1 c boiling)
- Pumpkin seeds (1 T)

What to Do:
- Combine the dry ingredients in your food processor until it is finely ground. Pour in the water and blend; slowly moving from low to high, until it smooth.
- Place in a bowl and top with extra coconut, sunflower seeds, and raisins.

Lunch: Low Carb Mexican Cauliflower Rice

Total Prep & Cooking Time: 15 minutes
Yields: 2 Servings

Nutrition Stats (one serving)
- Protein: 7.9 grams
- Net Carbs: 4.2 grams
- Fats: 18.3 grams
- Calories: 170

What to Use
- Cauliflower florets (3 C)
- Olive oil (1 T)
- Garlic cloves (4 minced)
- Jalapeno (1 finely chopped)
- Onion (1 small, finely chopped)
- Tomatoes (2 medium, finely chopped)
- Bell peppers (.75 c diced)
- Cumin powder (1 tsp.)
- Red chili powder (.5 tsp.)
- Coriander (1 T chopped)
- Salt (as desired)
- Cilantro (as desired)
- Avocados (1 sliced)

What to Do
- Process cauliflower florets and pulse till the cauliflower resembles small bits (like rice). Do not over process as it will turn mushy.
- Squish out the moisture from the cauliflower using paper towels
- Heat oil in a pan and toss onions, garlic and jalapenos. Stir fry till the onion is translucent and the garlic is fragrant.
- Toss in the tomatoes, cumin powder, paprika powder and salt to the pan. Cook the tomatoes for a few minutes till they soften. Add the diced bell peppers and cauliflower rice to the pan and mix well. Stir fry the cauliflower for 3-4 minutes till tender.
- Top with your favorite toppings and serve hot.

Dinner: Salmon with Spinach Sauce

Total Prep & Cooking Time: 130 minutes
Yields: 1 Serving

Nutrition Stats (one serving)
- Protein: 34 grams
- Net Carbs: 3.7 grams
- Fats: 56.4 grams
- Calories: 563

What to Use
- Salt (as desired)
- Pepper (as desired)
- Hollandaise sauce (1 serving)
- Ghee (2 T)
- Whipping cream (1 T)
- Spinach (1 large packet)
- Salmon fillet (1)

What to Do
- Heat up the oven to 400F. Drizzle some oil over the salmon and season. Place onto a tray and cook for 20 minutes.
- While that cooks, prepare the sauce. Wash your spinach and put it inside your spinner for salads to get rid of the water.
- Add half the ghee to the skillet and cook the spinach for 5 minutes. Add in the whipping cream.
- When salmon is done cooking, take it out of the oven and cool down.
- Pour the spinach sauce into a big bowl and top with the salmon. Pour the Hollandaise sauce on top before serving.

Day 12

Breakfast: Keto Omelet Wrap

Total Prep & Cooking Time: 10 minutes
Yields: 1 Serving

Nutrition Stats (one serving)
- Protein: 22 grams
- Net Carbs: 3.3 grams
- Fats: 29.2 grams
- Calories: 307

What to Use
- Salt (as desired)
- Pepper (as desired)
- Ghee (1 T)
- Onion (1 small)
- Chives (2 T chopped)
- Cream cheese (2 T)
- Smoked salmon (1 oz.)
- Avocado (.5 average)
- Eggs (3 large)

What to Do
- Crack eggs in a bowl add pepper and salt. Beat well.
- Mix cream cheese with chives. Slice smoked salmon. Cut the avocado in half and remove pit. Cut into slices. Heat ghee in a pan and add eggs. Don't cook the eggs too fast or they will end up tough. Cook until set well. Place omelet on a plate and spread on cream cheese.
- Add onion, avocado, and salmon. Fold to make a wrap. Enjoy.

Lunch: Buffalo Chicken Salad Sandwiches

Total Prep & Cooking Time: 30 minutes
Yields: 4 Servings

Nutrition Stats (one serving)
- Protein: 25 grams
- Net Carbs: 6.7 grams
- Fats: 35.7 grams
- Calories: 349

What to Use - Bun
- Baking powder (1 tsp)
- Eggs (4 beaten)
- Heavy cream (3.5 T)
- Golden flax meal (2.5 T)
- Coconut flour (2.5 T sifted)
- Butter (2 T)

What to Use - Chicken Salad
- Ranch dressing (4 T)
- Mayonnaise (3 T)
- Celery (2 T minced)
- Salt (.25 tsp)
- Garlic powder (.25 tsp)
- Celery seed (.25 tsp)
- Butter (3 T)
- Hot sauce (.3 c)
- Chicken (2 c cooked, shredded)

What to Do
- Heat oven to 400F.
- Grease 4 glass ramekins.
- In a bowl add all the bun ingredients and stir vigorously. Scrape sides and break up any clumps. Spoon batter equally into each ramekin. Bake for about 15 minutes until center is done. Take out of the oven and cool completely. Cut the buns in half. These can be toasted if desired.
- In a saucepan add, butter, salt, garlic powder, celery seed, hot sauce. Melt and stir to combine. Add cooked chicken and celery and stir. Take off the heat. Mix the mayonnaise and combine.

- To make the sandwiches, put .5 c chicken mixture on each bun. Top with ranch dressing. Serve and enjoy.

Dinner: Cheese Enchiladas

Total Prep & Cooking Time: 10 minutes
Yields: 6 Servings

Nutrition Stats (one serving)
- Protein: 27.2 grams
- Net Carbs: 5 grams
- Fats: 32 grams
- Calories: 376

What to Use – Enchilada Shells
- Cauliflower (3 c from one 16-oz. bag, frozen and thawed, drained, diced)
- Eggs (3)
- Mozzarella cheese (3 c), or Monterey Jack cheese

What to Use - Sauce
- Onion (.5 c, chopped)
- Garlic (2 large cloves, chopped and crushed)
- Chili powder (1 T)
- Oil (4 T, healthy oil)
- Oregano (1 tsp.)
- Pizza sauce (1 c)
- Cheddar cheese (2 c, shredded)
- Pepper Jack (2 c, shredded)
- Cumin (2 tsp)
- Salt (as desired)
- Pepper (as desired)

What to Do
- Preheat oven to 450F.
- Mix the cauliflower, cheese, and eggs.
- Put the mixture onto two cookie sheets in .3 c amounts, making 12 6-inch flat rounds.
- Bake each sheet for approximately 15 minutes or until the edges brown.
- Let cool. Then loosen them. Let set.

- Meanwhile, start making the sauce by chopping the onions and garlic cloves, and shredding the cheese.
- Add 4 T coconut oil to a skillet before placing it on top of a burner turned to a medium heat.
- Add in chili powder, garlic, and onion, garlic and let every cook for approximately 5 minutes.
- Mix in the tomato sauce and season as desired. Stir just until heated.
- Mix the cheeses.
- Get out a 9x13 casserole dish.
- Dredge each shell through the sauce and lay into the casserole dish golden side up.
- Put .25 c of the mixed cheddar and jack cheeses or of Monterey Jack cheese into each shell.

Day 13

Breakfast: Vegan Keto granola

Total Prep & Cooking Time: 10 minutes
Yields: 6 Servings

Nutrition Stats (one serving)
- Protein: 6.3 grams
- Net Carbs: 1.2 grams
- Fats: 18.2 grams
- Calories: 151

What to Use
- Sunflower seeds (.5 c)
- Hemp hearts (.75 c)
- Chia seeds (.25 c)
- Flax seeds (.5 c)
- Psyllium husk powder (2 T)
- Cinnamon (1 T)
- Liquid stevia (.25 tsp.)
- Salt (.5 tsp)
- Water (1 c)

What to Do
- Use parchment paper to line the baking sheet as the oven heats to 300F.
- Take your seeds and in a food processor, let them grind to relatively large chunks after which you shall take all the dry ingredients and mix completely.
- Slowly while stirring, add the water to the mixture until it forms a thick dough. Take the batter and lay it spread on your sheet for baking all the way uniform at a quarter of an inch in thickness.
- Let the batter bake in the oven for about 45 minutes.
- After this duration, break the granola up and let it bake more until it achieves a crunchy texture.
- Take it out of the oven and let it cool after which you can break into subsequently smaller pieces.

Lunch: Mango Coconut Chicken Bowls

Total Prep & Cooking Time: 40 minutes
Yields: 4 Servings

Nutrition Stats (one serving)
- Protein: 26.3 grams
- Net Carbs: 3.6 grams
- Fats: 29.6 grams
- Calories: 453

What to Use - Chicken
- Sweetened coconut (.25 c)
- Avocado (1 sliced)
- Brown rice (2 c cooked)
- Chicken breasts (4 sliced lengthwise in half)

What to Use - Marinade
- Salt (1 tsp.)
- Garlic cloves (2 minced)
- Sriracha (1 T)
- Honey (1 T)
- Lime juice (2 T)
- Olive oil (2 T)
- Mango (1 large)

What to Use - Salsa
- Cilantro (.25 C)
- Red pepper (.5 diced)
- Salt (.75 tsp.)
- Corn (1.5 c)
- Black beans (1 can drained)
- Red onion (1 diced)
- Lime juice (1 T)

What to Do
- Ensure your oven is preheated to 425F.
- Cook rice according to package instructions.
- In a blender, mix all of mango marinade ingredients together till combined.
- Marinate chicken in half of mango mixture 10 minutes.

- Mix together corn salsa ingredients.
- Place chicken on a baking tray and bake 15-20 minutes till golden in color.
- Slice chicken and place into bowls, along with additional mango sauce, corn salsa, topped with shredded coconut and cilantro. Place avocado on top.

Dinner: Seafood Stew

Total Prep & Cooking Time: 10 minutes
Yields: 8 Servings

Nutrition Stats (one serving)
- Protein: 42 grams
- Net Carbs: 8 grams
- Fats: 42 grams
- Calories: 310

What to Use
- Crushed tomatoes (28 oz.)
- Vegetable broth (4 c)
- White wine (0.5 c)
- Garlic (3 cloves, minced)
- Zucchini (0.5 lb., cut into bite-sized pieces)
- Summer squash (0.5 lb., cut into bite-sized pieces)
- Onion (0.5 medium, diced)
- Dried thyme (1 tsp.)
- Dried basil (1 tsp.)
- Dried cilantro (1 tsp.)
- Celery salt (0.5 tsp.)
- Salt (0.5 tsp.)
- Pepper (0.5 tsp.)
- Red pepper flakes (0.25 tsp.)
- Cayenne pepper (1 pinch)
- Seafood (2 lbs.)

What to Do
- Add all the ingredients except for the seafood into the slow cooker.
- On high, cook for 2 to 3 hours or low for 4-6 hours.
- On high, add the seafood and cook for another 30-60 minutes.

Day 14

Breakfast: Southwest Bacon Omelet

Total Prep & Cooking Time: 15 minutes
Yields: 1 Serving

Nutrition Stats (one serving)
- Protein: 22grams
- Net Carbs: 4 grams
- Fats: 60grams
- Calories: 630

What to Use
- Eggs (3 large)
- Bacon (4 strips)
- Onion (.5 small)
- Jalapeno (.25 c)
- Cheddar cheese (.25 c shredded)

What to Do
- Grill bacon in a skillet until cooked. Remove from the skillet and let it cool.
- Chop jalapeño and onion, then sauté in bacon grease. Remove from the heat and place with the bacon.
- Add olive oil to the pan in order to coat, then drain off the fat combination.
- Crack and scramble eggs then place in a pan. Allow to cook for a moment, then add all ingredients.
- Fold over omelet and let it cook for 1 minute on either side.
- Serve and enjoy!

Lunch: Green Bean Tapenade

Total Prep & Cooking Time: 20 minutes
Yields: 6 Servings

Nutrition Stats (one serving)
- Protein: 5 grams
- Net Carbs: 0.2 grams
- Fats: 18.4 grams
- Calories: 185

What to Use
- Pepper (as desired)
- Green beans (1.5 lbs. ends removed)
- Black olive tapenade (.5 c)
- Salt (as desired)

What to Do
- Allow a medium pot of water to come to a boil.
- Place the green beans and boil about 5 minutes.
- Once beans are done, strain and allow to dry.
- Toss with tapenade until well coated.
- Season with pepper and salt.
- Serve and enjoy!

Dinner: Keto Curry

Total Prep & Cooking Time: 10 minutes
Yields: 6 Servings

Nutrition Stats (one serving)
- Protein: 17.5 grams
- Net Carbs: 4.3 grams
- Fats: 26.1 grams
- Calories: 342

What to Use
- Chicken breasts (2 cut into bite size pieces)
- Red pepper (1 sliced)
- Bean sprouts (.25 c)
- Coconut milk (1 c)
- Mushrooms (.25 c chopped)
- Shirataki noodles (1 c)
- Red curry paste (as desired)
- Onion (1 sliced)
- Garlic (1 clove minced)
- Cilantro (as desired)

What to Use
- Sauté onions and chicken until chicken is almost finished.
- Add everything else aside from coconut milk and red curry paste.
- Add coconut milk and 3 tbsp of red curry paste, then cook over medium heat. Add seasonings as desired.
- When it boils, everything is done. Garnish with cilantro.

Conclusion

Thanks for making it through to the end of *Keto Diet For Beginners: Complete Beginner's Guide To The Ketogenic Diet With Delicious And Easy Recipes To Lose Weight And Eat Healthy Everyday*, let's hope it was informative and able to provide you with all of the tools you need to achieve your weight loss goals, whatever it is that they may be. Just because you've finished this book doesn't mean there is nothing left to learn on the topic, and expanding your horizons is the only way to find the mastery you seek.

Now that you have finished this book you have all the tools you need to get started with the keto diet as quickly and painlessly as possible. While you are no doubt likely ready and raring to go, it is important to keep in mind that you will have more luck if you give some thought to when you are going to make the transition to ketosis.

As it will be difficult for you body to make the change, it is important to choose a time in which you have the ability to relax and take it easy while your body gets its ketogenic processes online. Jumping in at the wrong time can make the transition far more difficult than it needs to be, opening up the potential for your keto diet journey to be over before it has properly begun. Remember, following the keto diet is a marathon, not a sprint, which means that slow and steady wins the race.

Finally, if you found this book useful in anyway, a review on Amazon is always appreciated!

Recipes Index In Alphabetical Order

Other Books By Julie Arden

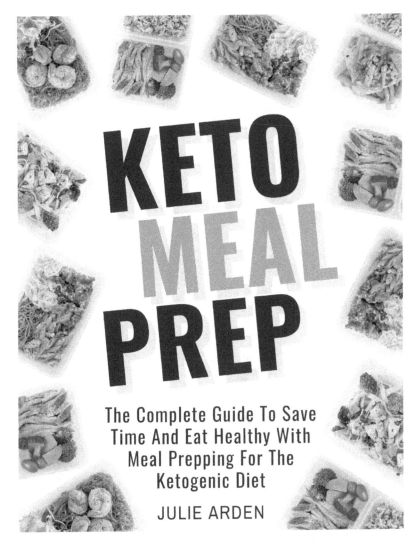

"Keto Meal Prep" by Julie Arden is available at Amazon.

CPSIA information can be obtained
at www.ICGtesting.com
Printed in the USA
LVHW080929161120
671799LV00014B/1193

9 781513 668321